YOGA SEQUENCING 101

A Beginners Guide To Flow From Amateur To Yogi

Almeida Jackov

Table Of Contents

INTRODUCTION TO YOGA SEQUENCING................. 3

UNDERSTANDING YOGA BASICS........................... 10

   Essential Yoga Equipment......................... 15

GETTING STARTED WITH YOGA SEQUENCING..... 18

BUILDING YOUR SEQUENCES................................ 29

YOGA SEQUENCES FOR COMMON CHALLENGES...
36

ADVANCED SEQUENCING TECHNIQUES................ 52

YOGA SEQUENCING FOR SPECIAL POPULATIONS..
61

PRACTICING SAFELY AND MINDFULLY.................. 72

INTEGRATING YOGA INTO YOUR DAILY LIFE........ 82

CONCLUSION.. 91

GLOSSARY OF YOGA TERMS................................. 98

INTRODUCTION TO YOGA SEQUENCING

Yoga sequencing is the art of arranging yoga poses in a purposeful order to create a balanced and effective practice. It involves structuring a series of yoga postures in a logical progression, taking into account factors such as breath, alignment, and energy flow. By thoughtfully sequencing yoga poses, practitioners can enhance physical strength, flexibility, and mental focus while promoting overall well-being.

What is Yoga Sequencing?

Yoga sequencing goes beyond simply stringing together poses randomly. It involves understanding the purpose and benefits of each pose and arranging them in a sequence that serves a specific intention or goal. This could be to energize the body, release tension, improve flexibility, build strength, or cultivate mindfulness.

At its core, yoga sequencing is about creating a holistic experience that addresses the needs of the body, mind, and spirit. It considers factors such as the balance between active and passive poses, the rhythm of breath, the alignment principles of yoga, and the individual abilities and limitations of practitioners.

Benefits of Yoga Sequencing for Beginners

For beginners, yoga sequencing offers numerous benefits that contribute to a fulfilling and sustainable practice:

1. Structured Progression: A well-designed sequence provides a structured progression from simple to more challenging poses, allowing beginners to gradually build strength, flexibility, and confidence in their practice.

2. Safe and Effective Practice: Proper sequencing ensures that beginners practice poses in a safe and anatomically sound manner, reducing the risk of injury and discomfort.

3. Improved Body Awareness: Following a sequence helps beginners develop greater body awareness as they learn to move mindfully and with intention through each posture.

4. Enhanced Learning Experience: By repeating poses in different sequences, beginners deepen their understanding of alignment, breath, and the subtle nuances of each pose.

5. Balanced Practice: Sequencing ensures a balanced practice that addresses all areas of the body, including strength, flexibility, balance, and mobility, promoting overall physical well-being.

6. Stress Relief and Relaxation: Thoughtfully curated sequences can help beginners release tension, calm the mind, and cultivate a sense of relaxation and inner peace.

7. Increased Confidence: Progressing through sequenced practices allows beginners to see tangible improvements in their abilities, boosting confidence and motivation to continue their yoga journey.

How to Use This Book

This book serves as a comprehensive guide to yoga sequencing specifically tailored for beginners. Here's how you can make the most of it:

1. Read the Introduction: Start by familiarizing yourself with the foundational concepts of yoga sequencing outlined in the introduction section.

2. Follow the Sequences: Explore the various sequences provided in the book, each designed to serve different goals and intentions. Begin with sequences labeled as suitable for beginners and gradually progress to more advanced practices as you gain experience.

3. Practice Mindfully: Pay close attention to the instructions provided for each pose and sequence. Focus on proper alignment, breath awareness, and listening to your body's cues to ensure a safe and effective practice.

4. Modify as Needed: Understand that every body is different, and it's essential to listen to your body's limitations and modify poses as needed. The book includes guidance on how to modify poses to suit your individual needs and abilities.

5. Stay Consistent: Establish a regular practice routine based on the sequences

provided in the book. Consistency is key to experiencing the full benefits of yoga sequencing.

6. Reflect and Adjust: Take time to reflect on your practice journey and adjust your approach as needed. As you gain experience, you may find that certain sequences resonate with you more than others, or you may feel ready to explore more challenging practices.

7. Seek Further Guidance: If you have questions or need further clarification on any aspect of yoga sequencing, don't hesitate to seek guidance from experienced yoga teachers or resources recommended in the book.

By following these guidelines, you can embark on a fulfilling yoga journey that brings balance, strength, and mindfulness into your life. Enjoy the process of exploration and self-discovery as you delve deeper into the transformative practice of yoga sequencing.

UNDERSTANDING YOGA BASICS

Yoga is a rich and ancient practice that encompasses physical postures, breath control, meditation, and philosophical teachings aimed at promoting holistic well-being. Understanding the basics of yoga lays the foundation for a meaningful and fulfilling practice.

Origins and Philosophy of Yoga

Yoga originated in ancient India thousands of years ago and has since evolved into a diverse system of practices with various philosophical and spiritual traditions. The word "yoga" is derived from the Sanskrit root "yuj," meaning to yoke or unite, symbolizing the union of body, mind, and spirit.

The philosophy of yoga is deeply rooted in ancient texts such as the Vedas, Upanishads, and the Bhagavad Gita. These texts outline the principles and pathways of yoga, including:

1. The Eight Limbs of Yoga: As outlined by the sage Patanjali in the Yoga Sutras, the eight limbs of yoga provide a comprehensive framework for ethical and spiritual living. They include ethical principles (yamas and niyamas), physical postures (asanas), breath control (pranayama), sense withdrawal (pratyahara), concentration (dharana), meditation (dhyana), and enlightenment (samadhi).

2. Paths of Yoga: There are various paths or approaches to yoga, each suited to different temperaments and goals. These paths include Karma Yoga (the path of selfless service), Bhakti Yoga (the path of devotion), Jnana Yoga (the path of knowledge), and Raja Yoga (the path of meditation).

3. The Concept of Oneness: At its core, yoga teaches that all beings are interconnected

and part of the universal consciousness. Through yoga practice, individuals seek to realize their inherent unity with all of creation.

Understanding the philosophical underpinnings of yoga provides practitioners with a deeper appreciation for the practice and its transformative potential.

Different Styles of Yoga

Yoga has evolved over time, giving rise to a multitude of styles and approaches tailored to diverse preferences and needs. Some of the most popular styles of yoga include:

1. Hatha Yoga: Hatha yoga is a broad term that encompasses any yoga practice that involves physical postures (asanas) and breath control (pranayama). It is often used interchangeably with "yoga" in the West and serves as the foundation for many modern yoga styles.

2. Vinyasa Yoga: Vinyasa yoga is characterized by flowing sequences of poses linked together by synchronized breath. It emphasizes smooth transitions between poses, creating a dynamic and meditative practice.

3. Iyengar Yoga: Developed by B.K.S. This style of yoga focuses on precise alignment and the use of props (such as blocks, straps, and bolsters) to support the body in poses. It is known for its attention to detail and therapeutic approach.

4. Ashtanga Yoga: Ashtanga yoga follows a specific sequence of poses, practiced in a vigorous and sequential manner, synchronizing breath with movement. It is a physically demanding practice that builds strength, flexibility, and endurance.

5. Kundalini Yoga: Kundalini yoga incorporates dynamic movements,

breathing techniques, chanting, and meditation to awaken the dormant energy (kundalini) believed to reside at the base of the spine. It aims to cultivate spiritual awareness and inner transformation.

6. Yin Yoga: Yin yoga focuses on passive, long-held poses designed to target the connective tissues of the body, such as ligaments, tendons, and fascia. It promotes relaxation, flexibility, and introspection.

7. Restorative Yoga: Restorative yoga uses props to support the body in gentle, passive poses, allowing for deep relaxation and stress relief. It is especially beneficial for promoting recovery and healing.

Each style of yoga offers unique benefits and appeals to different preferences and intentions. Exploring various styles can help practitioners discover the approach that resonates most deeply with them.

Essential Yoga Equipment

While yoga can be practiced with minimal equipment, certain props and accessories can enhance the practice and support proper alignment and comfort. Some essential yoga equipment includes:

1. Yoga Mat: A yoga mat provides cushioning and traction for practicing yoga poses on the floor. It helps prevent slipping and provides a comfortable surface for seated and lying poses.

2. Yoga Blocks: Blocks are used to support the body in poses where flexibility or strength is limited. They can be placed under the hands, feet, or hips to provide stability and extension.

3. Yoga Strap: A yoga strap is a useful tool for extending reach and improving alignment in poses where flexibility is

limited, such as forward bends and seated twists.

4. Yoga Bolster: Bolsters are firm, cylindrical cushions used to support the body in restorative poses, providing gentle elevation and relaxation.

5. Blanket: A blanket can be used for extra padding and warmth during relaxation poses and to support the body in seated or reclined positions.

6. Meditation Cushion: For seated meditation practice, a cushion or bolster can provide support and elevation to promote proper posture and comfort.

7. Yoga Towel: A yoga towel is handy for absorbing sweat and providing traction on the mat, especially during vigorous or heated yoga practices.

By investing in quality yoga equipment and props, practitioners can create a supportive and comfortable practice environment that enhances their yoga experience and promotes safety and alignment.

Understanding the basics of yoga, including its origins, philosophy, different styles, and essential equipment, provides a solid foundation for embarking on a transformative yoga journey. Whether you're a beginner or seasoned practitioner, cultivating awareness and appreciation for the underlying principles of yoga can deepen your practice and enrich your life.

GETTING STARTED WITH YOGA SEQUENCING

Yoga sequencing is the art of arranging yoga poses in a purposeful order to create a balanced and effective practice. Getting started with yoga sequencing involves preparing your space, incorporating warm-up exercises, practicing breathing techniques (pranayama), and exploring basic yoga poses (asanas) suitable for beginners.

Preparing Your Space

Creating a conducive environment for yoga practice is essential for maximizing the benefits of sequencing. Here are some tips for preparing your space:

1. Clearing Clutter: Choose a quiet, clutter-free area where you can move freely without distractions. Clearing the space of

clutter helps create a peaceful and calming atmosphere conducive to practice.

2. Setting the Mood: Consider dimming the lights or lighting candles to create a cozy ambiance. Playing soft music or nature sounds can further enhance the atmosphere and promote relaxation.

3. Gathering Props: Depending on your practice preferences and needs, gather any props or equipment you may need, such as a yoga mat, blocks, straps, and blankets. Having these props readily available ensures you can practice comfortably and safely.

4. Creating Sacred Space: Consider creating a small altar or sacred space where you can place meaningful objects such as candles, crystals, or images that inspire and uplift you. This space can serve as a focal point for intention setting and reflection during your practice.

By taking the time to prepare your space mindfully, you set the stage for a focused and enriching yoga experience.

Warm-up Exercises

Warm-up exercises are essential for preparing the body and mind for the main yoga practice. They help increase circulation, loosen tight muscles, and improve range of motion. Here are some common warm-up exercises to incorporate into your yoga sequencing:

1. Joint Mobilization: Begin by gently moving through a series of joint mobilization exercises to lubricate the joints and improve mobility. This can include neck circles, shoulder rolls, wrist circles, hip circles, knee circles, and ankle rotations.

2. Dynamic Stretches: Incorporate dynamic stretches to warm up major muscle groups and increase flexibility. Examples include

cat-cow stretches, spinal twists, side stretches, and leg swings.

3. Sun Salutations (Surya Namaskar): Sun salutations are a traditional sequence of yoga poses that provide a comprehensive warm-up for the entire body. They involve flowing through a series of poses, including mountain pose, forward fold, plank, upward-facing dog, and downward-facing dog, coordinated with breath.

4. Breath Awareness: Use the warm-up phase to cultivate breath awareness and synchronize movement with breath. Practice deep, diaphragmatic breathing (belly breathing) to calm the nervous system and center the mind.

By incorporating warm-up exercises into your yoga sequencing, you prepare your body and mind for the more intensive aspects of the practice, promoting safety and effectiveness.

Breathing Techniques (Pranayama)

Breath control, or pranayama, is an integral aspect of yoga practice. Pranayama techniques help regulate the breath, calm the mind, and enhance energy flow throughout the body. Here are some fundamental pranayama techniques for beginners:

1. Deep Belly Breathing (Diaphragmatic Breathing): Lie down on your back or sit in a comfortable position. Place one hand on your belly and the other on your chest. Inhale deeply through your nose, allowing your belly to rise as you fill your lungs with air. Exhale slowly through your nose, drawing your navel towards your spine. Repeat for several breaths, focusing on the expansion and contraction of your belly.

2. Ujjayi Breath (Victorious Breath): Ujjayi breath is a technique that involves slightly

constricting the back of the throat to create a soft, audible sound during breathing. Sit or stand with a tall spine. Inhale deeply through your nose, then exhale slowly through your nose while gently constricting the muscles at the back of your throat. Continue this rhythmic breathing pattern, focusing on the sound and sensation of the breath.

3. Alternate Nostril Breathing (Nadi Shodhana): Nadi Shodhana is a balancing pranayama technique that involves alternating between the left and right nostrils. Sit comfortably with your spine erect. Use your right thumb to close your right nostril and inhale through your left nostril. Then, close your left nostril with your ring finger and exhale through your right nostril. Inhale through your right nostril, then close it and exhale through your left nostril. Continue alternating nostrils for several breaths, maintaining a smooth and steady rhythm.

4. Kapalabhati (Skull Shining Breath): Kapalabhati is an energizing pranayama technique that involves rapid, forceful exhalations followed by passive inhalations. Sit with a tall spine and close your eyes. Take a deep inhalation through your nose, then forcefully exhale through your nose by contracting your abdominal muscles. Allow the inhalation to happen naturally without effort. Start with a slow pace and gradually increase speed as you become comfortable with the technique. After several rounds, return to normal breathing and observe the effects.

Practicing pranayama techniques cultivates mindfulness, reduces stress, and promotes overall well-being. Begin with simple techniques and gradually explore more advanced practices as you deepen your practice.

Basic Yoga Poses (Asanas) for Beginners

Basic yoga poses, or asanas, form the foundation of a yoga practice. They help develop strength, flexibility, balance, and body awareness. Here are some beginner-friendly yoga poses to include in your sequencing:

1. Mountain Pose (Tadasana): Stand tall with your feet hip-width apart, arms relaxed at your sides. Root down through your feet, engage your thighs, and lengthen your spine. Draw your shoulder blades down and back, and reach the crown of your head towards the sky. Hold the pose for several breaths, focusing on grounding and alignment.

2. Downward-Facing Dog (Adho Mukha Svanasana): Start on your hands and knees, with your wrists under your shoulders and knees under your hips. Spread your fingers

wide and press into your palms as you lift your hips towards the ceiling, forming an inverted V shape with your body. Keep your knees slightly bent and your heels reaching towards the floor. Lengthen your spine and draw your belly towards your thighs. Hold the pose for several breaths, feeling a stretch through the backs of your legs and spine.

3. Child's Pose (Balasana): Begin on your hands and knees, with your wrists under your shoulders and knees hip-width apart. Lower your hips back towards your heels as you reach your arms forward, resting your forehead on the mat. Allow your chest to melt towards the floor and your spine to lengthen. Take deep breaths into your back body, feeling a gentle stretch through your hips, spine, and shoulders.

4. Warrior I (Virabhadrasana I): Start in a standing position with your feet hip-width apart. Step your right foot back, keeping your toes pointing slightly outwards. Bend

your left knee, stacking it directly over your left ankle, and square your hips towards the front of the mat. Reach your arms overhead, palms facing each other, and gaze towards your fingertips.

In conclusion, getting started with yoga sequencing involves several key components that lay the foundation for a fulfilling and transformative practice. Preparing your space creates a supportive environment conducive to focus and relaxation. Incorporating warm-up exercises helps prepare the body and mind for the main practice, promoting safety and effectiveness. Exploring breathing techniques (pranayama) cultivates mindfulness, reduces stress, and enhances energy flow. Finally, practicing basic yoga poses (asanas) for beginners builds strength, flexibility, and body awareness.

By integrating these elements into your yoga sequencing journey, you embark on a path of self-discovery, growth, and holistic well-being. Whether you're new to yoga or an experienced practitioner, approaching your practice with mindfulness, intention, and reverence for its ancient roots allows you to tap into its profound transformative potential. As you continue to explore and deepen your practice, may you find joy, peace, and balance on your yoga journey.

BUILDING YOUR SEQUENCES

Building effective yoga sequences involves understanding the principles of sequencing and applying them creatively to create sequences tailored to specific goals and intentions. Whether you're designing a sequence for relaxation, strength, flexibility, or any other purpose, following these principles ensures a balanced and harmonious practice.

Principles of Sequencing

1. Warm-Up: Begin with gentle warm-up poses and movements to prepare the body for more intense postures. This may include joint mobilization exercises, dynamic stretches, and slow-paced movements to increase circulation and flexibility.

2. Progressive Flow: Sequence poses in a logical progression, moving from simpler to more challenging poses. This allows

practitioners to gradually build strength, flexibility, and confidence while minimizing the risk of injury.

3. Balanced Action: Create balance within the sequence by incorporating poses that target different muscle groups and movement patterns. Include a mix of forward bends, backbends, twists, lateral bends, and inversions to ensure a comprehensive practice.

4. Counterposing: Include counterposes to balance the effects of each pose and prevent muscle imbalances. For example, after a series of backbends, incorporate forward bends to release tension in the spine and counteract compression.

5. Breath Awareness: Coordinate movement with breath to create a fluid and meditative flow. Encourage practitioners to synchronize their breath with each

movement, using inhales to expand and exhales to release tension.

6. Alignment and Safety: Prioritize proper alignment and safety in each pose, offering clear instructions and modifications as needed. Emphasize stability and integrity in the joints to prevent strain and injury.

7. Transitions: Pay attention to the transitions between poses, ensuring they are smooth and fluid. Encourage practitioners to maintain mindfulness and awareness throughout the practice, even during transitions.

8. Rest and Integration: Incorporate periods of rest and integration throughout the sequence to allow practitioners to pause, reflect, and connect with their breath and body. Savasana (corpse pose) at the end of the practice provides an opportunity for deep relaxation and integration of the benefits of the practice.

By following these principles, you can create yoga sequences that are safe, effective, and transformative, supporting practitioners in their journey towards holistic well-being.

Sample Sequences for Different Goals

1. Relaxation Sequence:
   - Begin in a comfortable seated position, focusing on deep, diaphragmatic breathing.

   - Move into gentle warm-up poses such as Cat-Cow, Child's Pose, and Thread the Needle.

   - Transition into soothing poses such as Legs-Up-The-Wall, Reclining Bound Angle Pose, and Supine Twist.

   - Conclude with a relaxation pose such as Savasana, allowing practitioners to surrender into deep relaxation and stillness.

2. Strength Sequence:
   - Start with dynamic warm-up poses such as Sun Salutations (Surya Namaskar) to warm up the body and build heat.

   - Incorporate strength-building poses such as Plank, Warrior Poses, and Boat Pose to challenge the muscles and build endurance.

   - Include balancing poses such as Tree Pose and Warrior III to improve stability and focus.

   - Conclude with grounding poses such as Bridge Pose and Corpse Pose to release tension and restore energy.

3. Flexibility Sequence:
   - Begin with gentle warm-up poses such as Cat-Cow, Downward-Facing Dog, and Standing Forward Bend to stretch and lengthen the muscles.

- Move into deeper stretches such as Low Lunge, Extended Triangle Pose, and Pigeon Pose to target specific muscle groups and increase flexibility.

- Incorporate passive stretches such as Reclining Hand-to-Big-Toe Pose and Happy Baby Pose to release tension and improve range of motion.

- Conclude with a relaxation pose such as Savasana to integrate the benefits of the practice and allow the body to relax fully.

4. Balance Sequence:
   - Start with grounding poses such as Mountain Pose and Tree Pose to establish stability and focus.

- Incorporate challenging balancing poses such as Eagle Pose, Half Moon Pose, and Dancer's Pose to improve balance and coordination.

- Include core-strengthening poses such as Boat Pose and Plank variations to support stability and control.

- Conclude with a seated meditation or breathing exercise to center the mind and cultivate inner balance.

These sample sequences provide a starting point for creating yoga practices tailored to specific goals and intentions. Feel free to modify and adapt them based on individual preferences, abilities, and needs. As you explore and experiment with sequencing, remember to stay connected to the principles of yoga and the needs of your practitioners, cultivating a practice that honors the body, mind, and spirit.

YOGA SEQUENCES FOR COMMON CHALLENGES

Yoga offers effective solutions for addressing common challenges such as stress, back pain, poor posture, and difficulty sleeping. By incorporating specific poses and practices into your yoga sequences, you can help alleviate these issues and promote overall well-being.

Yoga for Stress Relief

Stress has become a prevalent issue in today's fast-paced world, impacting physical, mental, and emotional health. Yoga offers a holistic approach to stress relief by combining movement, breathwork, and mindfulness practices. Here's a sample yoga sequence for stress relief:

1. Child's Pose (Balasana): Begin in a kneeling position with your big toes together and knees apart. Sit back on your heels and

fold forward, resting your forehead on the mat. Extend your arms forward or alongside your body. Breathe deeply into your lower back and allow your body to relax completely.

2. Cat-Cow Stretch: Transition to a tabletop position with your wrists under your shoulders and knees under your hips. Inhale as you arch your back, dropping your belly towards the floor and lifting your gaze (Cow Pose). Exhale as you round your spine, tucking your chin towards your chest and drawing your navel towards your spine (Cat Pose). Flow smoothly between these two poses with each breath for several rounds.

3. Standing Forward Bend (Uttanasana): From tabletop position, tuck your toes and lift your hips up and back into Downward-Facing Dog. Walk your feet towards your hands at the top of the mat, coming into a forward fold. Allow your upper body to relax completely, releasing

tension from your neck and shoulders. You can bend your knees as much as needed to maintain a comfortable stretch in your hamstrings.

4. Legs-Up-The-Wall (Viparita Karani): Lie on your back with your hips close to a wall. Extend your legs up the wall and rest your arms by your sides. Close your eyes and focus on deep, slow breaths. Allow gravity to gently release tension from your legs and lower back. Stay in this pose for 5-10 minutes, breathing deeply and allowing your body to relax fully.

5. Corpse Pose (Savasana): Transition to Savasana by lying flat on your back with your arms by your sides and your legs extended. Close your eyes and let your body sink into the mat. Scan your body for any remaining areas of tension and consciously release them with each exhale. Stay in Savasana for 5-10 minutes, allowing yourself to rest deeply and restore your energy.

This sequence focuses on gentle stretches, relaxation poses, and mindful breathing to release physical and mental tension, promoting a sense of calm and relaxation.

Yoga for Back Pain

Back pain is a common ailment that can be caused by various factors, including poor posture, muscle imbalances, and tightness. Yoga can help alleviate back pain by improving spinal alignment, strengthening core muscles, and increasing flexibility. Here's a sample yoga sequence for back pain relief:

1. Cat-Cow Stretch: Begin in a tabletop position with your wrists under your shoulders and knees under your hips. Inhale as you arch your back, dropping your belly towards the floor and lifting your gaze (Cow Pose). Exhale as you round your spine, tucking your chin towards your chest and

drawing your navel towards your spine (Cat Pose). Flow smoothly between these two poses with each breath for several rounds to warm up the spine and increase mobility.

2. Downward-Facing Dog (Adho Mukha Svanasana): From tabletop position, tuck your toes and lift your hips up and back, coming into an inverted V shape. Press firmly into your hands and feet, lengthening your spine and lifting your sitting bones towards the ceiling. Keep a slight bend in your knees and focus on lengthening your spine and releasing tension from your back.

3. Low Lunge (Anjaneyasana): Step your right foot forward between your hands and lower your left knee to the mat. Keep your right knee stacked over your right ankle and your fingertips on the floor or on blocks for support. Engage your core and lengthen your spine as you lift your chest and gaze forward. Hold the pose for several breaths,

feeling a gentle stretch in the front of your left hip and thigh.

4. Child's Pose (Balasana): Transition to Child's Pose by sitting back on your heels and folding forward, resting your forehead on the mat and extending your arms forward or alongside your body. Focus on deep, slow breaths into your lower back, allowing your body to relax completely and release tension.

5. Supine Twist: Lie on your back with your arms extended to the sides in a T shape. Bend your knees and draw them towards your chest. Exhale as you lower your knees to the right side, keeping both shoulders grounded on the mat. Gaze towards your left hand and breathe deeply into the twist, feeling a gentle stretch in your spine and outer hip. Hold for several breaths, then repeat on the other side.

6. Corpse Pose (Savasana): Conclude the sequence by transitioning to Savasana. Lie flat on your back with your arms by your sides and your legs extended. Close your eyes and allow your body to sink into the mat, releasing any remaining tension. Stay in Savasana for 5-10 minutes, focusing on deep relaxation and allowing your body to integrate the benefits of the practice.

This sequence targets the muscles of the back, hips, and core, promoting flexibility, strength, and alignment to alleviate back pain and prevent future discomfort.

Yoga for Better Posture

Poor posture can lead to a variety of health issues, including neck and back pain, decreased mobility, and compromised breathing. Yoga offers effective strategies for improving posture by strengthening the muscles that support proper alignment and increasing body awareness. Here's a sample yoga sequence for better posture:

1.   Mountain Pose (Tadasana): Begin standing at the top of your mat with your feet hip-width apart and parallel. Ground down through your feet and engage your thighs. Lengthen your spine, draw your shoulder blades down and back, and reach the crown of your head towards the sky. Allow your arms to hang by your sides with your palms facing forward. Take several deep breaths, feeling tall and aligned in Mountain Pose.

2. Chair Pose (Utkatasana): From Mountain Pose, inhale as you sweep your arms overhead, palms facing each other. Exhale as you bend your knees and sit back as if you're sitting in an imaginary chair. Keep your weight in your heels and your knees stacked over your ankles. Engage your core and lengthen your spine, lifting your chest and gaze. Hold the pose for several breaths,

feeling the strength and stability in your legs and core.

3. Warrior II (Virabhadrasana II): Step your right foot back and rotate your body to face the long edge of your mat. Extend your arms parallel to the floor, with your right arm reaching back and your left arm reaching forward. Bend your left knee to stack it directly over your left ankle, keeping your right leg straight and strong. Square your hips towards the side of the mat and gaze over your left fingertips. Hold the pose for several breaths, feeling grounded and centered.

4. Reverse Warrior (Viparita Virabhadrasana): From Warrior II, inhale as you reach your left arm up towards the sky, lengthening your left side body. Keep your left knee bent and your right arm resting lightly on your right leg. Gaze towards your lifted hand or down towards the mat,

depending on your neck's comfort. Feel the stretch along your left side body and the strength in your legs. Hold the pose for several breaths, focusing on maintaining stability and openness.

5. Extended Triangle Pose (Utthita Trikonasana): Straighten your left leg and reach your left arm forward, coming into a straight line from your fingertips to your left heel. Hinge at your left hip and lower your left hand to your shin, ankle, or a block, keeping your right arm extended towards the sky. Align your shoulders and stack them vertically over your hips. Gaze towards your right fingertips or up towards your right hand, depending on your neck's comfort. Feel the lengthening and opening through your side body and the engagement in your legs. Hold the pose for several breaths, then repeat on the other side.

6. Seated Forward Fold (Paschimottanasana): Sit on the mat with

your legs extended in front of you. Flex your feet and engage your quadriceps. Inhale as you lengthen your spine, then exhale as you hinge at your hips and fold forward over your legs. Reach for your shins, ankles, or feet, depending on your flexibility. Keep your spine long and avoid rounding your back. Relax your neck and shoulders, and breathe deeply into the stretch. Hold the pose for several breaths, feeling a gentle release in your hamstrings and lower back.

7. Bridge Pose (Setu Bandhasana): Lie on your back with your knees bent and your feet hip-width apart, flat on the mat. Press your feet into the mat as you lift your hips towards the ceiling. Interlace your hands underneath your body and roll your shoulders onto the mat. Engage your glutes and thighs to lift your hips higher, creating a straight line from your shoulders to your knees. Keep your neck relaxed and breathe deeply into your chest. Hold the pose for

several breaths, feeling a gentle opening in your chest and shoulders.

8. Corpse Pose (Savasana): Conclude the sequence by transitioning to Savasana. Lie flat on your back with your arms by your sides and your legs extended. Close your eyes and allow your body to sink into the mat. Release any remaining tension and surrender to deep relaxation. Stay in Savasana for 5-10 minutes, focusing on your breath and allowing your body and mind to integrate the benefits of the practice.

This sequence focuses on strengthening the muscles that support proper posture, stretching tight muscles, and improving body awareness to promote better alignment and balance. Practicing regularly can help correct postural imbalances and prevent future discomfort or injury.

Yoga for Relaxation and Sleep

In today's fast-paced world, many people struggle with stress and insomnia, making it difficult to relax and get restful sleep. Yoga offers gentle and effective practices to calm the nervous system, quiet the mind, and prepare the body for deep relaxation and sleep. Here's a sample yoga sequence for relaxation and better sleep:

1. Seated Meditation: Begin in a comfortable seated position, either cross-legged on the floor or sitting on a cushion or block. Close your eyes and take a few deep breaths to center yourself. Allow your attention to focus on your breath, letting go of any thoughts or distractions. Spend a few minutes in silent meditation, cultivating a sense of inner calm and presence.

2. Supine Spinal Twist (Supta Matsyendrasana): Lie on your back with your arms extended to the sides in a T shape. Bend your knees and draw them towards your chest. Exhale as you lower

your knees to the right side, keeping both shoulders grounded on the mat. Gaze towards your left hand and breathe deeply into the twist, feeling a gentle release in your spine and hips. Hold for several breaths, then repeat on the other side.

3. Legs-Up-The-Wall (Viparita Karani): Sit close to a wall with one hip touching the wall. Lie on your back and swing your legs up the wall, resting your heels against the wall and your arms by your sides. Close your eyes and focus on deep, slow breaths. Allow your body to relax completely as you surrender to gravity. Stay in this pose for 5-10 minutes, feeling a sense of lightness and ease.

4. Supported Bridge Pose (Setu Bandhasana): Place a yoga block or bolster underneath your sacrum and lower back. Lie back on the prop with your knees bent and feet flat on the floor. Allow your arms to rest by your sides with your palms facing up.

Close your eyes and relax into the support of the prop. Breathe deeply into your chest and belly, feeling a sense of grounding and relaxation. Hold the pose for several minutes, allowing your body to soften and release tension.

5. Corpse Pose (Savasana): Conclude the sequence by transitioning to Savasana. Lie flat on your back with your arms by your sides and your legs extended. Close your eyes and take several deep breaths, allowing your body to relax completely. Scan your body for any remaining areas of tension and consciously release them with each exhale. Stay in Savasana for 10-15 minutes, surrendering to deep relaxation and allowing yourself to drift into a peaceful sleep.

This sequence focuses on gentle stretches, restorative poses, and calming breathwork to soothe the nervous system, quiet the mind, and prepare the body for deep relaxation and sleep. Practicing these poses regularly before bedtime can help promote better sleep quality and overall well-being.

Incorporating these yoga sequences into your regular practice can provide effective solutions for common challenges such as stress, back pain, poor posture, and difficulty sleeping. Whether you're looking to relax, alleviate discomfort, or improve your overall health and well-being, yoga offers a holistic approach to addressing these issues and promoting optimal physical, mental, and emotional wellness.

ADVANCED SEQUENCING TECHNIQUES

Advanced sequencing techniques in yoga involve going beyond basic poses and simple transitions to create more dynamic, challenging, and innovative sequences. These techniques incorporate elements such as props, pose modifications, and dynamic flow to deepen the practice and enhance its effectiveness. Let's explore some advanced sequencing techniques in detail:

Incorporating Props into Your Practice

Yoga props are valuable tools that can support alignment, deepen stretches, and enhance the overall yoga experience. Incorporating props into your practice allows you to modify poses, adapt sequences to individual needs, and explore new dimensions of alignment and awareness.

Here are some common props and how to use them effectively:

1. Yoga Blocks: Yoga blocks are versatile props that can be used to modify poses, provide support, and increase accessibility. They can be placed under the hands, feet, or sitting bones to bring the floor closer to you or provide stability in challenging poses. For example, in Triangle Pose (Trikonasana), placing a block under the bottom hand can help maintain alignment and stability while reaching towards the floor.

2. Yoga Straps: Yoga straps are useful for increasing flexibility, improving alignment, and accessing deeper stretches. They can be looped around the feet, hands, or body to extend reach and support in poses where flexibility is limited. For example, in the Seated Forward Fold (Paschimottanasana), looping a strap around the feet and gently pulling can help lengthen the spine and deepen the stretch without straining.

3. Yoga Bolsters: Yoga bolsters are firm cushions that provide support and comfort in restorative poses and deep stretches. They can be used to elevate the hips, support the spine, or cushion the body in reclining poses. For example, in Supported Bridge Pose (Setu Bandhasana), placing a bolster under the sacrum can elevate the hips and release tension in the lower back.

4. Yoga Blankets: Yoga blankets are versatile props that can be used for padding, support, and warmth during practice. They can be folded or rolled to provide cushioning under sensitive areas such as knees, elbows, or hips. For example, in Child's Pose (Balasana), placing a folded blanket under the forehead can provide support and help release tension in the neck and shoulders.

By incorporating props into your practice, you can customize your yoga experience to suit your body's needs, enhance alignment and stability, and explore new possibilities in your practice.

Modifying Poses for Different Levels

Modifying poses for different levels allows practitioners to adapt the practice to their individual abilities, limitations, and goals. Whether you're a beginner, intermediate, or advanced practitioner, there are ways to modify poses to make them more accessible or challenging. Here are some strategies for modifying poses:

1. Use Props: Props can be used to modify poses by providing support, stability, and alignment. For example, using a block under the hand or a strap to extend reach can make poses more accessible for beginners or those with limited flexibility.

2. Adjust Alignment: Paying attention to alignment cues and making subtle adjustments can make a significant

difference in the experience of a pose. For example, in Warrior II (Virabhadrasana II), aligning the front knee directly over the ankle and stacking the shoulders over the hips creates a stable and balanced foundation.

3. Offer Variations: Provide variations of poses to accommodate different levels of flexibility, strength, and experience. For example, offering a modified version of a pose with bent knees or a gentler approach can make it more accessible for beginners or those with injuries.

4. Focus on Breath and Awareness: Encourage practitioners to focus on their breath and body awareness rather than striving for a specific shape or depth in a pose. Emphasize the importance of listening to the body, honoring its limitations, and practicing with mindfulness and compassion.

By modifying poses for different levels, you can create inclusive and supportive yoga sequences that meet the needs of all practitioners, regardless of their experience or ability.

Creating Dynamic Flow Sequences

Dynamic flow sequences involve moving dynamically from one pose to another in a fluid and continuous manner, synchronizing movement with breath. These sequences create heat, build strength, improve flexibility, and cultivate mindfulness as practitioners flow through a series of poses. Here are some tips for creating dynamic flow sequences:

1. Focus on Breath: Coordinate movement with breath to create a smooth and rhythmic flow. Encourage practitioners to inhale as they move into expansive poses and exhale as they move into contracting poses. Linking breath with movement helps create a

meditative state and enhances the flow of energy throughout the body.

2. Sequence Poses Creatively: Arrange poses in a logical and purposeful order, moving seamlessly from one pose to the next. Consider the relationship between poses and how they complement each other in terms of alignment, action, and intention. Include a variety of poses that target different muscle groups and movement patterns to create a balanced and well-rounded practice.

3. Offer Transitions: Pay attention to transitions between poses and offer creative ways to flow between them. Explore different transitions such as vinyasas, chaturangas, and dynamic movements that challenge balance, coordination, and strength. Smooth and fluid transitions keep the energy flowing and maintain the rhythm of the practice.

4. Include Peak Poses: Incorporate peak poses or challenging poses that serve as focal points for the sequence. Build up to these poses gradually, preparing the body and mind with appropriate warm-up poses and modifications. Peak poses offer an opportunity for practitioners to challenge themselves, explore their edge, and experience a sense of accomplishment.

By creating dynamic flow sequences, you can offer practitioners a transformative and engaging yoga experience that builds strength, flexibility, and mindfulness, leaving them feeling energized, centered, and empowered.

In conclusion, advanced sequencing techniques in yoga offer a rich and diverse array of tools and strategies for deepening the practice and expanding its potential. By incorporating props, modifying poses, and creating dynamic flow sequences, you can tailor the practice to meet the needs of individual practitioners, support their growth and development, and foster a sense of connection, exploration, and transformation on the mat.

YOGA SEQUENCING FOR SPECIAL POPULATIONS

Yoga is a versatile practice that can be adapted to meet the needs of various populations, including seniors, pregnant women, and children. Sequencing yoga practices for special populations requires careful consideration of their unique physical, mental, and emotional needs, as well as any specific contraindications or limitations they may have. Here's a detailed exploration of yoga sequencing for seniors, prenatal yoga sequencing, and yoga for children:

Yoga for Seniors

Seniors can benefit greatly from practicing yoga, as it helps improve flexibility, balance, strength, and overall well-being. When sequencing yoga practices for seniors, it's important to focus on gentle movements, mindful breathing, and poses that support joint health and mobility. Here are some key considerations for yoga sequencing for seniors:

1. Warm-Up: Begin with gentle warm-up exercises to prepare the body for movement and increase circulation. This may include joint mobilization exercises, gentle stretches, and slow-paced movements to loosen tight muscles and joints.

2. Chair Yoga: Incorporate chair yoga poses to make the practice accessible for seniors with mobility issues or balance concerns. Chair yoga allows practitioners to perform modified versions of traditional yoga poses while seated or using the chair for support.

3. Balance Poses: Include balance poses to help seniors improve stability and reduce the risk of falls. Poses such as Tree Pose, Warrior III, and Eagle Pose can help strengthen the muscles of the legs and core while improving balance and coordination.

4. Flexibility Exercises: Focus on poses that target areas of stiffness and tightness, such as the hips, shoulders, and spine. Gentle stretches and restorative poses like Cat-Cow, Seated Forward Fold, and Supine Twist can help improve flexibility and range of motion.

5. Breathing Techniques: Integrate breathwork (pranayama) into the practice to promote relaxation, reduce stress, and increase mindfulness. Encourage seniors to practice slow, deep breathing techniques such as diaphragmatic breathing or alternate nostril breathing.

6. Mindfulness and Meditation: Include periods of mindfulness and meditation to help seniors cultivate presence, awareness, and inner peace. Guided meditation, body scan practices, and visualization exercises can help seniors connect with their breath

and body, reduce anxiety, and improve mental clarity.

By sequencing yoga practices with these considerations in mind, seniors can enjoy the many benefits of yoga while honoring their bodies and abilities.

Prenatal Yoga Sequencing

Prenatal yoga offers numerous benefits for pregnant women, including relief from discomfort, preparation for childbirth, and connection with the baby. When sequencing yoga practices for pregnant women, it's essential to prioritize safety, comfort, and modifications that accommodate the changing needs of the body during pregnancy. Here's a guide to prenatal yoga sequencing:

1. Warm-Up: Begin with a gentle warm-up to mobilize the spine, hips, and pelvis and prepare the body for movement. This may

include Cat-Cow stretches, gentle pelvic tilts, and seated hip circles to release tension and increase circulation.

2. Modified Poses: Adapt traditional yoga poses to accommodate the changing anatomy and needs of pregnant women. Modify poses such as twists, deep backbends, and inversions to ensure safety and comfort. Use props such as bolsters, blankets, and blocks to provide support and stability in poses.

3. Pelvic Floor Exercises: Incorporate pelvic floor exercises to strengthen the pelvic floor muscles and prepare for childbirth. Kegel exercises, pelvic tilts, and squatting poses can help improve pelvic floor function and stability, reducing the risk of pelvic floor dysfunction.

4. Hip-Opening Poses: Focus on hip-opening poses to relieve tension and discomfort in the hips and pelvis. Poses

such as Pigeon Pose, Butterfly Pose, and Wide-Legged Forward Fold can help stretch and release tight muscles, improve flexibility, and create space for the baby.

5. Breathing and Relaxation Techniques: Teach breathing techniques and relaxation exercises to help pregnant women manage stress, reduce anxiety, and connect with their breath and body. Practices such as diaphragmatic breathing, ujjayi breath, and guided relaxation can promote relaxation, calmness, and mental clarity.

6. Bonding with Baby: Incorporate poses and practices that foster a sense of connection with the baby in the womb. Gentle movements, visualization exercises, and mindful awareness of the baby's presence can help pregnant women cultivate a deeper bond with their growing baby and enhance the prenatal experience.

By sequencing prenatal yoga practices with these considerations in mind, pregnant women can safely and effectively support their physical, emotional, and spiritual well-being throughout pregnancy.

Yoga for Children

Yoga offers numerous benefits for children, including improved flexibility, strength, coordination, and emotional regulation. When sequencing yoga practices for children, it's important to make the practice fun, engaging, and age-appropriate, incorporating playful movements, imaginative themes, and interactive activities. Here's how to sequence yoga practices for children:

1. Playful Warm-Up: Begin with a playful warm-up to energize the body and engage the imagination. Incorporate fun movements such as animal poses (e.g., Cat-Cow, Downward-Facing Dog), dynamic

stretches, and silly movements that encourage children to move and explore their bodies.

2. Themed Sequences: Create themed sequences based on children's interests, such as animals, nature, superheroes, or fairy tales. Use storytelling, visual aids, and props to bring the theme to life and make the practice exciting and engaging for children.

3. Partner Poses: Include partner poses and group activities to promote teamwork, cooperation, and social interaction. Partner poses such as Partner Tree Pose, Partner Boat Pose, and Partner Forward Fold encourage children to work together, communicate, and support each other in their practice.

4. Breathing Games: Teach children simple breathing exercises through interactive games and activities. Breathing games such

as "Bubble Breath" (inhaling deeply and exhaling through pursed lips to blow imaginary bubbles) or "Birthday Candle Breath" (inhaling deeply and exhaling slowly to blow out a pretend birthday candle) help children develop awareness of their breath and cultivate relaxation and focus.

5. Mindfulness and Relaxation: Introduce mindfulness and relaxation practices to help children calm their minds and bodies and reduce stress and anxiety. Guided visualizations, progressive muscle relaxation, and mindfulness activities such as "Mindful Eating" (slowly savoring a piece of food with full attention) help children develop mindfulness skills and emotional resilience.

6. Creative Expression: Encourage creative expression through art, music, and movement. Allow children to express themselves creatively through drawing,

dancing, singing, or storytelling, integrating these activities into the yoga practice to foster self-expression, confidence, and self-awareness.

By sequencing yoga practices with these considerations in mind, children can experience the joy, benefits, and transformative power of yoga in a playful and supportive environment.

In conclusion, yoga sequencing for special populations requires thoughtful consideration of their unique needs, abilities, and preferences. Whether sequencing yoga practices for seniors, pregnant women, or children, it's essential to prioritize safety, comfort, and inclusivity, adapting the practice to meet individuals where they are and support their physical, mental, and emotional well-being. Through mindful and compassionate yoga sequencing, practitioners of all ages and abilities can experience the transformative power of yoga and cultivate a deeper connection with themselves and others.

PRACTICING SAFELY AND MINDFULLY

Practicing yoga safely and mindfully is essential to prevent injuries, promote physical and mental well-being, and deepen the connection with oneself. By cultivating awareness of the body, breath, and mind, practitioners can navigate their yoga practice with greater ease, grace, and self-care. Here's an exploration of injury prevention tips, listening to your body, and the importance of rest and recovery in yoga:

Injury Prevention Tips

Injury prevention is paramount in yoga to ensure a safe and sustainable practice. By following these tips, practitioners can reduce the risk of injuries and maintain a healthy relationship with their bodies:

1. Warm-Up Properly: Begin each yoga session with a thorough warm-up to prepare

the body for movement and prevent strain or injury. Gentle movements, dynamic stretches, and breathwork can help increase circulation, loosen tight muscles, and lubricate the joints.

2. Focus on Alignment: Pay attention to proper alignment in each pose to avoid unnecessary strain on the joints and muscles. Align the body carefully, engage the core, and distribute weight evenly to maintain stability and integrity in the poses.

3. Use Props Wisely: Props such as blocks, straps, and bolsters can provide support, stability, and alignment assistance in yoga poses. Use props mindfully to modify poses, accommodate limitations, and prevent overstretching or strain.

4. Avoid Overexertion: Listen to your body and honor its limits. Avoid pushing yourself too hard or forcing your body into uncomfortable or painful positions. Instead,

practice with awareness, compassion, and sensitivity to your body's needs.

5. Modify Poses as Needed: Modify poses as needed to accommodate injuries, limitations, or physical conditions. Adapt poses with the guidance of a qualified instructor to ensure safety and prevent exacerbating existing issues.

6. Stay Hydrated: Drink plenty of water before, during, and after your yoga practice to stay hydrated and support optimal physical function. Proper hydration is essential for maintaining joint lubrication, muscle function, and overall well-being.

By following these injury prevention tips, practitioners can create a safe and supportive environment for their yoga practice, allowing them to reap the benefits of yoga without risking injury or harm.

Listening to Your Body

Listening to your body is a foundational principle of yoga that encourages practitioners to tune into their physical sensations, emotions, and intuition. By cultivating body awareness and practicing mindfulness, practitioners can develop a deeper understanding of their bodies' needs and limitations. Here's how to listen to your body in yoga:

1. Tune into Sensations: Pay attention to physical sensations in the body, such as tightness, discomfort, or pain. Notice how each movement and pose feels and adjust accordingly to find a balance between effort and ease.

2. Practice Mindful Awareness: Cultivate mindful awareness of the present moment by focusing on the sensations of the breath, the rhythm of the body, and the quality of thoughts and emotions. Mindfulness helps bring attention to the body's signals and

promotes a sense of presence and connection.

3. Honor Your Limits: Respect your body's limits and boundaries by practicing within your comfort zone. Avoid comparing yourself to others or pushing yourself beyond your capabilities. Instead, embrace your unique strengths and challenges and practice with self-compassion and acceptance.

4. Modify Poses as Needed: Modify poses as needed to accommodate your body's needs and limitations. Listen to any signals of discomfort or strain and adapt poses with props, variations, or adjustments to ensure safety and comfort.

5. Take Breaks When Necessary: Take breaks as needed during your practice to rest, hydrate, and recharge. Listen to your body's signals of fatigue, exhaustion, or

discomfort and honor the need for rest and recovery.

6. Cultivate Self-Compassion: Approach your practice with kindness, patience, and self-compassion. Be gentle with yourself, especially on days when you're feeling tired, stressed, or unmotivated. Remember that yoga is not about perfection but about self-discovery and self-care.

By listening to your body with curiosity, compassion, and openness, you can deepen your yoga practice, prevent injuries, and cultivate a deeper connection with yourself.

The Importance of Rest and Recovery

Rest and recovery are essential components of a balanced yoga practice that support physical, mental, and emotional well-being. In our fast-paced society, it's easy to overlook the importance of rest and prioritize constant activity and productivity.

However, rest is crucial for rejuvenating the body, calming the mind, and restoring energy levels. Here's why rest and recovery are essential in yoga:

1. Muscle Repair and Growth: Rest allows the body to repair damaged tissues, replenish energy stores, and promote muscle growth and recovery. During rest periods, the body undergoes processes such as protein synthesis, which rebuilds and strengthens muscle fibers damaged during exercise.

2. Prevention of Overtraining: Overtraining occurs when the body is subjected to excessive physical stress without adequate time for recovery. Overtraining can lead to fatigue, decreased performance, increased risk of injury, and burnout. Rest days and periods of active recovery are essential for preventing overtraining and maintaining optimal performance.

3. Stress Reduction: Rest and relaxation techniques such as meditation, deep breathing, and gentle movement promote the activation of the parasympathetic nervous system, which induces a state of relaxation and reduces the body's stress response. Restorative yoga practices are particularly effective for promoting relaxation and stress reduction.

4. Mental Clarity and Focus: Rest allows the mind to unwind, recharge, and reset, promoting mental clarity, focus, and cognitive function. Quality sleep and rest periods enhance memory consolidation, problem-solving abilities, and overall cognitive performance.

5. Injury Prevention: Adequate rest and recovery time allow the body to heal and repair itself, reducing the risk of overuse injuries, muscle imbalances, and chronic fatigue. Incorporating rest days into your yoga practice helps prevent burnout and

promotes longevity and sustainability in your practice.

6. Emotional Well-Being: Rest and relaxation are essential for promoting emotional well-being, resilience, and balance. Taking time to rest and engage in activities that nourish the soul, such as spending time in nature, connecting with loved ones, or engaging in creative pursuits, helps replenish energy levels and foster a sense of inner peace and contentment.

By prioritizing rest and recovery as integral parts of your yoga practice, you can optimize physical performance, enhance mental clarity, and cultivate a deeper sense of well-being and vitality.

In conclusion, practicing yoga safely and mindfully requires attention to injury prevention, listening to your body, and honoring the importance of rest and recovery. By incorporating these principles into your yoga practice, you can create a supportive and sustainable approach to yoga that promotes holistic well-being, resilience, and self-care. Through mindful awareness and compassionate self-reflection, practitioners can navigate their yoga practice with greater ease, grace, and joy, cultivating a deeper connection with themselves and the world around them.

INTEGRATING YOGA INTO YOUR DAILY LIFE

Yoga is not just a physical practice but a way of life that offers numerous benefits for the body, mind, and spirit. Integrating yoga into your daily life allows you to cultivate mindfulness, reduce stress, and promote overall well-being. Here's how you can incorporate yoga into your daily routine:

Establishing a Regular Practice Routine

1. Set Realistic Goals: Determine how often you want to practice yoga each week and set realistic goals based on your schedule and commitments. Start with a manageable number of days per week, such as two or three, and gradually increase as you build consistency and confidence.

2. Create a Dedicated Space: Designate a quiet, clutter-free space in your home where

you can practice yoga comfortably. Set up a yoga mat, props, and any other accessories you may need to support your practice. Having a dedicated space can help create a sense of ritual and make it easier to commit to your practice.

3. Choose a Convenient Time: Schedule your yoga practice at a time that works best for you and fits into your daily routine. Whether it's first thing in the morning, during your lunch break, or in the evening before bed, choose a time when you're least likely to be interrupted and can't fully immerse yourself in the practice.

4. Start Small: Begin with short, manageable practice sessions, such as 15-20 minutes, and gradually increase the duration and intensity as you progress. Focus on consistency rather than intensity, and listen to your body's needs as you build strength, flexibility, and endurance.

5. Be Flexible: Be flexible and adaptable with your practice routine, especially during busy or challenging times. If you're unable to practice at your usual time or for the full duration, try to squeeze in a shorter session or practice mindfulness and breathing exercises throughout the day to stay connected to your practice.

6. Stay Accountable: Hold yourself accountable to your practice by setting reminders, tracking your progress, and seeking support from friends, family, or online communities. Share your goals and challenges with others who can offer encouragement, motivation, and accountability along the way.

By establishing a regular practice routine and integrating yoga into your daily life, you can experience the transformative benefits of yoga on a consistent basis, leading to greater physical, mental, and emotional well-being.

Using Yoga for Stress Management

1. Practice Mindful Breathing: Incorporate mindful breathing exercises into your daily routine to reduce stress and promote relaxation. Practice deep, diaphragmatic breathing, or try techniques such as ujjayi breath, alternate nostril breathing, or belly breathing to calm the nervous system and induce a state of relaxation.

2. Engage in Gentle Movement: Take short breaks throughout the day to engage in gentle movement and stretching exercises to release tension and alleviate stress. Practice simple yoga poses such as Cat-Cow, Forward Fold, or Child's Pose to stretch tight muscles, improve circulation, and promote relaxation.

3. Practice Yoga Nidra: Incorporate yoga nidra, or yogic sleep, into your daily routine to promote deep relaxation and

rejuvenation. Set aside time each day to lie down in a comfortable position and listen to a guided yoga nidra meditation to release stress, tension, and fatigue from the body and mind.

4. Cultivate Mindfulness: Practice mindfulness throughout your day by bringing awareness to your thoughts, emotions, and sensations in the present moment. Engage in activities such as walking meditation, mindful eating, or body scan exercises to cultivate mindfulness and reduce stress.

5. Connect with Nature: Spend time outdoors in nature to reduce stress, boost mood, and promote overall well-being. Take a walk in the park, go for a hike in the mountains, or simply sit outside and soak up the sun and fresh air to rejuvenate the mind and body.

6. Nourish Yourself: Take care of your physical and emotional needs by nourishing yourself with healthy food, adequate sleep, and meaningful connections with others. Practice self-care activities such as journaling, reading, or spending time with loved ones to recharge and replenish your energy reserves.

By incorporating yoga into your daily life as a tool for stress management, you can cultivate greater resilience, inner peace, and well-being, even in the midst of life's challenges and uncertainties.

Incorporating Yoga into Other Activities

1. Yoga at Work: Incorporate yoga into your workday by practicing desk yoga or chair yoga exercises to relieve tension, improve posture, and boost energy levels. Take short breaks throughout the day to stretch, breathe, and reset your mind and body.

2. Yoga and Fitness: Complement your existing fitness routine with yoga to enhance flexibility, balance, and mobility. Incorporate yoga poses and sequences that target specific areas of the body affected by your primary form of exercise, such as running, cycling, or weightlifting.

3. Yoga and Sports: Use yoga as a cross-training tool to support your athletic performance and prevent injuries. Incorporate yoga poses and movements that mimic the demands of your sport, such as hip openers for runners, shoulder stretches for swimmers, or core strengtheners for golfers.

4. Yoga and Recreation: Integrate yoga into your recreational activities such as hiking, biking, or swimming to enhance your overall enjoyment and performance. Practice yoga poses and breathing techniques before and

after your recreational activities to warm up, cool down, and recover more effectively.

5. Yoga and Creativity: Use yoga as a tool to enhance creativity, inspiration, and self-expression. Practice yoga poses and meditation techniques that stimulate the flow of energy and creativity in the body and mind, such as hip openers, heart openers, or visualization exercises.

6. Yoga and Relationships: Share your love of yoga with others by practicing yoga with friends, family, or partners. Practice partner yoga poses, acro yoga, or group yoga classes to deepen your connections, foster trust, and create shared experiences with others.

By integrating yoga into other activities and aspects of your life, you can enrich your overall experience, deepen your practice, and reap the benefits of yoga both on and off the mat.

In conclusion, integrating yoga into your daily life is a powerful way to cultivate greater mindfulness, reduce stress, and enhance overall well-being. By establishing a regular practice routine, using yoga for stress management, and incorporating yoga into other activities, you can experience the transformative effects of yoga in all areas of your life. Through mindful awareness, self-care, and intentionality, you can create a balanced and holistic approach to living that supports your physical, mental, and emotional health and vitality.

CONCLUSION

As you come to the end of your yoga journey, it's essential to take a moment to reflect on how far you've come, acknowledge your progress, and celebrate your achievements. The practice of yoga is not just about physical postures; it's a journey of self-discovery, growth, and transformation that unfolds both on and off the mat. In this conclusion, we'll reflect on your yoga journey and offer final words of encouragement to support you on your path.

Reflecting on Your Yoga Journey

1. Personal Growth: Take a moment to reflect on how yoga has impacted your life and contributed to your personal growth and development. Notice how your body, mind, and spirit have evolved throughout your practice, and recognize the positive changes and insights you've gained along the way.

2. Challenges and Triumphs: Reflect on the challenges you've faced and the triumphs you've experienced during your yoga journey. Acknowledge the moments of struggle and adversity as valuable opportunities for growth and learning, and celebrate the moments of breakthrough and accomplishment.

3. Mind-Body Connection: Consider how your relationship with your body has evolved through your yoga practice. Notice the increased awareness, sensitivity, and connection you've developed with your body's sensations, rhythms, and needs, and honor the wisdom that arises from deepening this mind-body connection.

4. Emotional Resilience: Reflect on how yoga has supported your emotional well-being and resilience in navigating life's ups and downs. Notice how the practice of mindfulness, breathwork, and self-reflection

has helped you cultivate greater inner peace, equanimity, and acceptance in the face of challenges.

5. Community and Connection: Reflect on the relationships and connections you've cultivated through your yoga practice. Celebrate the sense of community, support, and camaraderie you've found within your yoga community and the bonds you've formed with fellow practitioners on the shared journey of self-discovery and growth.

6. Gratitude and Appreciation: Take a moment to express gratitude and appreciation for the teachers, mentors, and guides who have inspired and supported you along your yoga journey. Recognize the impact they've had on your practice and the profound influence they've had on your life.

As you reflect on your yoga journey, honor the unique path you've traveled and the wisdom you've gained along the way.

Embrace the lessons learned, the challenges overcome, and the growth experienced, knowing that your yoga journey is a lifelong exploration of self-discovery and transformation.

Final Words of Encouragement

1. Trust the Process: Trust in the process of yoga and the wisdom of your own inner guidance. Remember that growth takes time, patience, and perseverance, and that each step along the journey is an opportunity for learning, healing, and growth.

2. Embrace Imperfection: Embrace imperfection and let go of the need for perfection in your practice. Recognize that yoga is not about achieving the perfect pose or attaining a certain level of mastery but about embracing the journey with humility, curiosity, and compassion.

3. Listen to Your Heart: Listen to the whispers of your heart and follow your intuition as you navigate your yoga journey. Trust in your inner wisdom to guide you towards practices, teachings, and experiences that resonate with your deepest truth and highest potential.

4. Be Gentle with Yourself: Be gentle with yourself and practice self-compassion as you encounter challenges, setbacks, and moments of self-doubt. Cultivate a nurturing and supportive inner dialogue that fosters self-love, self-acceptance, and self-care.

5. Celebrate Your Progress: Celebrate your progress, no matter how small or incremental it may seem. Acknowledge the growth, the breakthroughs, and the moments of courage and resilience that have brought you to this point on your journey.

6. Stay Open and Curious: Stay open and curious to the infinite possibilities that await you on your yoga journey. Approach each practice with a beginner's mind, a sense of wonder, and a willingness to explore and discover new dimensions of yourself and the world around you.

As you continue on your yoga journey, may you be guided by the light of your own inner wisdom, supported by the love and encouragement of your community, and inspired by the boundless potential that resides within you. Remember that the true essence of yoga lies not in the poses you practice but in the depth of presence, connection, and awareness you bring to each moment of your life. With an open heart and a steadfast commitment to growth and self-discovery, may you continue to shine brightly and illuminate the path for others on their journey of awakening and transformation.

In closing, know that the journey of yoga is a lifelong adventure, a sacred pilgrimage of self-discovery and self-realization that unfolds with each breath, each step, and each moment of presence and awareness. May your yoga journey be filled with love, light, and blessings, and may you continue to shine brightly as you walk the path of awakening and liberation. Namaste.

GLOSSARY OF YOGA TERMS

Yoga is a rich and diverse practice with its own unique terminology that can sometimes be confusing for beginners. This glossary aims to provide clarity by defining common yoga terms, concepts, and Sanskrit terminology frequently used in yoga classes, literature, and discussions. Understanding these terms can deepen your knowledge and enhance your yoga practice.

1. Asana: A Sanskrit term that refers to yoga poses or postures. Asanas are physical exercises that cultivate strength, flexibility, and balance, as well as promote relaxation and mindfulness.

2. Pranayama: The practice of breath control or regulation. Pranayama techniques involve conscious manipulation of the breath to enhance vitality, increase mental clarity, and promote relaxation.

3. Vinyasa: A flowing sequence of yoga poses coordinated with breath. Vinyasa yoga emphasizes fluid movement, smooth transitions between poses, and synchronization of breath with movement.

4. Hatha Yoga: A traditional style of yoga that focuses on physical postures (asanas) and breath control (pranayama). Hatha yoga practices typically include a combination of static poses, dynamic movements, and breathwork.

5. Surya Namaskar: Also known as Sun Salutation, Surya Namaskar is a dynamic sequence of yoga poses performed in a flowing sequence. It is traditionally practiced in the morning to greet the sun and energize the body and mind.

6. Drishti: A focal point or gaze point used during yoga practice to promote concentration, balance, and inner awareness. Each yoga pose has a specific

drishti, which helps align the body and mind.

7. Mantra: A sacred sound, word, or phrase repeated during meditation or chanting practices to focus the mind, cultivate inner peace, and invoke spiritual energy. Mantras are often recited in Sanskrit and hold symbolic significance.

8. Mudra: A symbolic hand gesture or seal used in yoga and meditation practices to channel energy, enhance concentration, and facilitate deeper states of awareness. Mudras are believed to stimulate specific energy pathways in the body.

9. Chakra: In yogic philosophy, chakras are subtle energy centers located along the spine that correspond to different aspects of physical, emotional, and spiritual well-being. There are seven main chakras, each associated with specific qualities and characteristics.

10. Namaste: A traditional Indian greeting that is commonly used at the end of a yoga class. Namaste is a gesture of respect and gratitude that acknowledges the divine light within each individual.

11. Om: A sacred sound and spiritual symbol often chanted at the beginning or end of yoga classes, meditation practices, and rituals. Om represents the primordial sound of the universe and the eternal essence of existence.

12. Yogi/Yogini: A practitioner of yoga. The term "yogi" traditionally refers to a male practitioner, while "yogini" refers to a female practitioner. However, these terms are often used interchangeably to describe anyone who engages in the practice of yoga.

13. Bandha: A yogic lock or energy seal that is engaged during yoga poses and breathwork to direct and control the flow of

prana (life force energy) in the body. There are three main bandhas: Mula Bandha (root lock), Uddiyana Bandha (abdominal lock), and Jalandhara Bandha (throat lock).

14. Savasana: Also known as Corpse Pose, Savasana is a relaxation pose practiced at the end of a yoga class. It involves lying flat on the back with the arms and legs extended, allowing the body to relax completely and integrate the benefits of the practice.

15. Yamas and Niyamas: The ethical and moral guidelines of yoga, as outlined in Patanjali's Yoga Sutras. The Yamas are principles of self-restraint and social conduct, while the Niyamas are principles of self-discipline and personal observance.

16. Prana: The Sanskrit term for life force energy or vital energy. Prana is believed to permeate all living beings and is responsible for sustaining physical, mental, and spiritual

well-being. Pranayama practices aim to cultivate and balance prana in the body.

17. Aumkara: Another term for the sacred sound of Om, representing the three aspects of cosmic consciousness: creation, preservation, and dissolution. Aumkara is often chanted as a mantra to invoke spiritual presence and connect with the divine.

18. Sadhana: A spiritual practice or discipline undertaken with dedication and devotion to cultivate self-awareness, inner peace, and spiritual growth. Sadhana may include yoga, meditation, chanting, or other rituals performed regularly with sincerity and intention.

19. Guru: A spiritual teacher or guide who imparts wisdom, knowledge, and guidance to students on the path of yoga and self-realization. The word "guru" is derived

from Sanskrit and means "dispeller of darkness."

20. Karma: The law of cause and effect or the principle of action and reaction in the universe. Karma is the cumulative result of one's actions, thoughts, and intentions, which shape one's destiny and future experiences.

By familiarizing yourself with these yoga terms, you can deepen your understanding of the practice and enhance your ability to communicate and connect with fellow practitioners and teachers. Whether you're a beginner or an experienced yogi, integrating these terms into your vocabulary can enrich your yoga journey and foster a deeper sense of connection with the ancient wisdom and traditions of yoga.